SLEEP TOOLS

The Secrets Of Restful and Restorative Sleep

by Keith Scott-Mumby MD, MB ChB, HMD, PhD

Sleep Tools: Secrets Of Restful and Restorative Sleep

Publishers: Mother Whale Inc.

8550 W Charleston Blvd. Suite #102-160, Las Vegas, NV 89117

ISBN: 978-1-7334785-3-3

Library of Congress registration number applied for.

Printed in the United States of America

Book Design: Dragos Balasoiu

Illustrations by: Oliver Scott-Mumby

Disclaimer

Sleep Quotes

"A good laugh and a long sleep are the best cures in the doctor's book."
— Irish proverb

"I tried counting sheep so I can fall asleep but that got boring, so I started talking to the shepherd instead."
— Anonymous

"Laugh and the world laughs with you, snore and you sleep alone."
— Anthony Burgess, *Inside Mr. Enderby*

"Man is a genius when he is dreaming."
— Akira Kurosawa, Japanese Film Director

"Sleep is like a cat: It only comes to you if you ignore it."
— Gillian Flynn, *Gone Girl*

"Dear sleep, I'm sorry we broke up this morning. I want you back!"
— Anonymous

"No civilized person goes to bed the same day he gets up."
— Richard Harding Davis, American Journalist

"I love sleep. My life has the tendency to fall apart when I'm awake, you know?"
— Ernest Hemingway, American Author

"No wonder Sleeping Beauty looked so good...she took long naps, never got old, and didn't have to do anything but snore to get her Prince Charming."
— Olive Green, Author

"I'm so good at sleeping that I can do it with my eyes closed."
— Anonymous

"Happiness is waking up, looking at the clock and finding that you still have two hours left to sleep."
— Charles M. Schulz, American Cartoonist

Contents

Part 1. The Secrets of Restful Restorative Sleep

Sleep engineering is a term invented by Penny Lewis, a sleep scientist and professor of psychology at Cardiff University (UK). It seems we need to engineer better sleeping. We need to take control of our sleep habits and get wise at it.

Sleep deprivation can measurably shorten your life. It's poor math to claim an extra 2-hours wakefulness a day, if you live 12 – 15 years less! Work it out...

The fact is, one in 3 of us suffers from poor sleep, with stress, computers and taking work home often blamed. However, the cost of all those sleepless nights is more than just bad moods and a lack of focus.

More than 70 types of sleep disorders exist. The most common problems are insomnia (difficulty falling or staying asleep), obstructive sleep apnea (disordered breathing that causes multiple awakenings), various movement syndromes (unpleasant sensations that prompt night fidgeting), and narcolepsy (extreme sleepiness or falling asleep suddenly during the day).

[Harvard Health Publishing Harvard Medical School: https://www.health.harvard.edu/ newsletter_article/sleep-and-mental-health

Many effects of a lack of sleep, such as feeling grumpy and not working at your best, are well known. But did you know that sleep deprivation can also have profound consequences on your physical health?

Continuing poor sleep puts you at risk of serious medical conditions, including obesity, heart disease and diabetes – and it shortens your life expectancy. It's now clear that a solid night's sleep is essential for a long and healthy life. [from the NHS website, UK]

In the famous "Whitehall II Study," into the lives and health of civil servants, British researchers discovered less than five hours of sleep *doubled the risk of death from cardiovascular disease.*

Thing is that sleep deprivation leads to serious inflammation throughout the body and inflammation is the number one ager, whether as depression, Alzheimer's disease, obesity, arteriosclerosis, diabetes or even cancer.

That's not all: research led by the Surrey Sleep Research Centre (UK) found that people who were subjected to sleep deprivation for a week underwent changes at a molecular level that could affect their well-being.

Sleeping fewer than six hours for several nights in a row affects hundreds of genes responsible for keeping us in good health.

[SOURCES: Dijk, D. PNAS, published online Feb. 25, 2013. Professor Adrian Williams, professor of sleep medicine, King's College, London. Professor Jim Horne, Sleep Research Centre, Loughborough University, England]

The important Sleep Heart Health Study observed that, in a large sample of US men and women, sleeping for five hours or less per night increased the odds of type II diabetes by a whopping 251%!

[Tuomilehto H, Peltonen M, Partinen M, Seppa J, Saaristo T, Korpi-Hyovalti E, et al. Sleep duration is associated with an increased risk for the prevalence of type 2 diabetes in middle-aged women—the FIN-D2D survey. Sleep Med. 2008;9(3):221–227]

Even too much sleep isn't good. Those who sleep nine or more hours have a 79% increased odds of type II diabetes and an 88% increased odds of pre-diabetes, compared to those who habitually slept just 7-8 hours.

The details emerging make sleep loss an inevitable disaster. As another example, a Mexican study of sleep deprived individuals showed damage to the important blood-brain barrier. That allows toxins to enter the brain which should not and for which there is no detox mechanism in the brain. [https://www.sciencedaily.com/releases/2014/06/140610101316.htm]

Make no mistake, sleep is a crucial health parameter.

This book is to help you get started on holistic sleep remedies, meaning sleep aids that do NOT include sleep medications such as Ambien and Lunesta. OTC sleep remedies, while less dangerous, are generally anti-histamines and have very limited benefits.

Understanding Your Sleep Cycles

Take a moment to be sure you understand this concept, we'll be referring to it again. The table herewith shows how we cycle through sleep patterns each night...

There are four stages of sleep and we cycle through each. Stages 1 and 2 are REM sleep, so-called (from random eye movements, which characterize that level of sleep).

A Typical 8 Hour Sleep Cycle

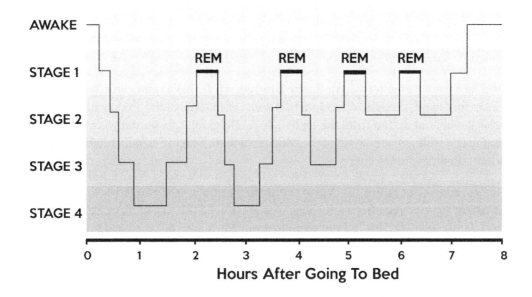

Hours After Going To Bed

In the US, stages 3 and 4 are combined to form what is lumped together as "deep sleep". In the rest of the world, the stage 3 and 4 terminology is used. It takes a full cycle to go down from stages 1 and 2, to deep sleep, and back up. There are five sleep cycles per night, making a total of 7 ½ to 8 hours.

Study the chart carefully and you will see that the first two sleep cycles are quite deep. After that they become shallower.

What we do know now is that the first part of a sleep cycle is about restoration and repair. There are no random eye movements in this phase (non-REM sleep). The brain waves at this time are slow and rhythmical, like breathing. These cycles have to do with processing short-term memory and converting it to long-term.

Conclusion? You need to be in bed well before midnight and fast asleep for maximum brain health. 10.30 pm. is a good bedtime, even though most people stay up later than that!

What About Afternoon Napping and Siesta?

For years I've been pointing out that taking an afternoon snooze has good science! It improves mental (cognitive) function, slows aging and extends memory. There is a whole raft of physiological benefits.

Taking a nap after lunch, the so-called siesta, is a widespread indulgence in hotter climes. Business is resumed when the sun has lost some of its power and continues through the coolness of the evening.

I lived for years in southern Spain in the late 1990s (Marbella) and can attest to the benefits first hand, though I speculate that some of that may have to do with sleeping off the alcohol imbibition from the night before! Drinking substantially is almost universal in the stifling hot climate of the Mediterranean, a factor usually totally ignored by ignorant dietetics "researchers".

There's science to back this up. A 2007 study of 23,000 cases from Greece showed that taking a nap in the afternoon considerably reduced the risk of heart attacks (37% fewer). Unfortunately, this did not seem to apply to women but they had fewer heart attacks anyway, in this particular study.

Researchers found that napping every day produced better results than doing it occasionally (only a 12% reduction). This is an important study because the notably lower incidence of coronary artery disease has always been attributed to diet – the so-called "Mediterranean Diet". It may be that researchers have been looking in the wrong direction. Maybe the siesta habit is the REAL secret of the Mediterranean "diet" success?

The Greek study covered 5 years from 1994 to 1999 and was conducted in 10 European countries. The participants were categorized as:

- never taking naps
- those taking midday naps occasionally and
- those napping often or daily

Naps were categorized as more than 30 minutes or less than 30 minutes. Taking daily naps of 30 minutes or more definitely helped health and survival.

The researchers compensated for other factors which might cloud the issue, such as physical activity, body mass index, smoking habit and, of course, diet itself.

What this seems to be telling us is that short naps are great for reducing stress on a daily basis and we all know the dangers of stress. There is considerable evidence that it causes short and long-term damage to health, including provoking heart disease and cancer.

Stress also destroys relationships and reduces productivity. Benjamin Franklin may have known this instinctively. He had a sleep-pattern characterized by periodic napping and he was very productive! [Arch Intern Med. 2007;167:296-301]

"Only mad dogs and Englishmen go out in the midday sun". It's actually a slight misquote from a line in a song by Noël Coward, which he got from an earlier piece by that most Indian of all English writers, Rudyard Kipling. Kipling once described the delirium produced by the sun in India, observing that only "mad dogs and Englishmen go out in the noonday sun". Coward used Kipling's line in the tune, without the word "only".

Scientific support for the benefits of a siesta time have continued over the years.

Afternoon Napping is Linked To Better Mental Agility

A 2020 study weighed in, with new data suggesting that taking a regular afternoon nap may be linked to better mental agility. The study, looking at over 2,000 of an older Chinese demographic, was published in the online journal General Psychiatry. [Relationship between afternoon napping and cognitive function in the ageing Chinese population, General Psychiatry, DOI: 10.1136/gpsych-2020-100361]

Basically, siesta seems to be associated with better locational awareness, verbal fluency, and working memory.

Longer life expectancy and the associated neurodegenerative changes that accompany it, raise the prospect of dementia, with around 1 in 10 people over the age of 65 affected in the developed world.

As people age, their sleep patterns change, with afternoon naps becoming more frequent. But research published to date hasn't reached any consensus on whether afternoon naps might help to stave off cognitive decline and dementia in older people or whether they might be a symptom of dementia.

To investigate this further, researchers took 2214 ostensibly healthy individuals aged at least 60 and resident in several large cities around China, including Beijing, Shanghai, and Xian.

In all, 1534 took a regular afternoon nap, while 680 didn't. All participants underwent a series of health checks and cognitive assessments, including the Mini Mental State Exam (MMSE), which checks for dementia.

The average length of night time sleep was around 6.5 hours in both groups.

For this paper, afternoon naps were defined as periods of at least five consecutive minutes of sleep, but no more than 2 hours, and taken after lunch—classic siesta time! Participants were asked how often they napped during the week; this ranged from once a week to every day.

The dementia screening tests included 30 items that measured several aspects of cognitive ability, and higher function, including visuo-spatial skills, working memory, attention span, problem solving, locational awareness and verbal fluency.

Interestingly, the MMSE cognitive performance scores were significantly higher among the nappers than they were among those who didn't nap. And there were significant differences in locational awareness, verbal fluency, and memory.

Of course studies like this don't prove cause and effect. Taking afternoon naps may not be the reason that some individuals scored better. It may simple be that individuals in good shape regularly felt the need for some "catch up" shuteye. But it still means there is something going on: what is it about those individuals that leads them to nap regularly, perhaps intuitively?

The nappers have something going for them!

One theory is that inflammation is a mediator between mid-day naps and poor health outcomes; inflammatory chemicals have an important role in sleep disorders, note the researchers.

Sleep regulates the body's immune response and napping is thought to be an evolved response to inflammation; people with higher levels of inflammation also nap more often, explain the researchers.

It comes down to what I have been saying for decades: sleep is the most powerful and healthful restorative there is. Your body cannot rest and regenerate, if you don't give it chance!

Nothing heals in the presence of inflammation. Fact!

You Snooze You Win

This is the title of a piece in the journal *Scientific American* (2002): new research, it says, indicates that morning sleep and afternoon naps aid mental and physical learning. Scientists have known for some time that sleep can improve the brains acquisition of new facts and skills, but its effect on previously learned knowledge was not known. But the position is quickly changing, starting with two landmark studies in July 2002, published in the journals *Neuron* and *Nature Neuroscience*. Both suggest that snoozing can reverse "burnout" from information overload and improve motor skill development.

In the first study, Sara Mednick of Harvard University investigated the role of sleep in perceptual learning. She and her team trained subjects to report the direction of colored bars superimposed on other lines on a computer screen. Their performance progressively worsened throughout the day. If the researchers allowed individuals to nap for 30 minutes, however, the deterioration halted; a one-hour snooze enabled performance to bounce back to initial morning levels.

Upon reaching a certain threshold, the brain seems to prevent the absorption of new information in order to allow the data already there to be committed to memory during slumber. Apparently, the deep, delta-wave sleep that occurs in even short naps allows recently learned information to be processed and the mind refreshed.

In the second study, internationally-known sleep scientist Matthew Walker and his collaborators, looked at the effects of sleep on motor skills. Subjects were taught to punch a certain sequence of keys, and they practiced the task for some time. But 12 hours later that same day, their speed and accuracy did not significantly improve. When the team retested them the next morning, after a good nights sleep, however, their performance improved markedly. The improvement directly related to what is known as stage 2 non-rapid eye movement sleep (see chart, page 3).

"This is the part of a good nights sleep that many people will cut short by getting up early in the morning," Walker cautions.

These findings may help answer the question: why infants sleep so much. Nobody has to learn more, or faster, than growing infants. They exist in a famine of information and live through a hunger for knowledge.

"Perhaps in the future a typical day at the office will start later and include a power nap," says Rachel Moeller, author of the SA article!

[https://www.scientificamerican.com/article/you-snooze-you-win-learni/]

So napping/siesta is good medicine. BUT NOT FOR MORE THAN ABOUT A HALF HOUR, OTHERWISE YOU RISK DISRUPTING YOUR BODY CLOCK.

The Real Value Of Yawning

Before we get started on sleep in earnest, here is some fascinating new science telling us what yawning is really all about (from an original essay by my friend and fellow health publisher Lee Euler: www.awakeningfromalzheimers.com)

For the longest time, the act of yawning puzzled medical researchers. Yawning seems commonplace and insignificant – you feel tired, you yawn. You see somebody else yawn, you yawn. You get bored, you yawn.

But why? What does yawning actually achieve?

The problem researchers faced was to figure out a definitive biological purpose for yawning. When they did, they discovered that every yawn actually helps the brain function better and remain more alert. It's almost counter-intuitive. Here's the surprising research.

Researchers in Switzerland found that yawning forms part of what's called the "thermoregulatory" system of the brain. It's controlled by a part of the brain called the hypothalamus, which regulates body temperature. [https://pubmed.ncbi.nlm.nih.gov/11896042/]

So, say researchers, a basic function of yawning is to lower the temperature of brain tissue. Lee Euler described this as your brain's "air conditioner", which is amusing!

One of the first clues about the brain-cooling function of yawns was the fact that in spring, as temperatures warm, people tend to yawn more. But then, as the body adjusts to the warmer temperatures, our yawning rate goes down.

Another clue is the discovery that brain tissue is consistently warmer than the blood flowing through the body. And when you yawn, as the muscles of the jaw open your mouth and contract, extra amounts of cooling blood course through your head – like the coolant that flows through a car engine radiator, to keep it from over-heating.

Plus, your sinuses also flex during a yawn. That allows for more cooling through the thin walls of the sinus as extra, cooler air, enters your head. [https://www.ncbi.nlm.nih.gov/pmc/articles/PMC3534187/]

So, in the same way that a cool breeze blowing across your face when you're tired can help you stay more awake when you're fatigued, the cooling action of a yawn can also boost your alertness.

My wife notices that when I have been working hard (meaning writing and using my mind strenuously), my head feels somewhat hot. That's not surprising. And probably why a dip on the pool during the excess heat of the day is very restorative to the intellect!

And along with this cooling action, researchers in Switzerland say that a yawn and the muscular contractions that go with it also boost circulation of the cerebrospinal fluid. That increased flow helps to clear the brain of natural chemicals such as adenosine (a neurotransmitter) and prostaglandin D(2) (a hormone), that are both linked to sleepiness. [https://pubmed.ncbi.nlm.nih.gov/23813685/]

Why Are Yawns Infectious?

As you've probably noticed, the act of yawning is contagious. If you see somebody else yawn, you're more likely to yawn. However, research in Italy demonstrates that not all yawns are equally contagious. Perhaps not surprisingly, the yawns of your closest family and friends are more catching than the yawns of strangers. [https://www.ncbi.nlm.nih.gov/pmc/articles/PMC7147458/]

Along with that, men's yawns elicit the yawns of other people more than female yawns do, while women are generally more likely than men to start yawning when other people yawn.

Interestingly, the bigger your brain, the longer your yawns. More brain tissue means you have more brain cells that need cooling – kind of like the way a large limo or SUV needs a bigger cooling system than a tiny Smartcar, says Lee Euler.

This also holds true for animals. A study on dogs shows that dogs with bigger heads and brains yawn for longer periods of time than small dogs with smaller heads.

One final yawning tip: If you're in an important meeting and you're trying to fend off the impolite urge to yawn, make sure to keep breathing through your nose. Air taken in through your nostrils and sinuses will cool your brain more than air that enters through your mouth and may make it easier to resist a yawn. [https://pubmed.ncbi.nlm.nih.gov/19657685/]

So, best advice is: if you want to yawn, don't fight it. Go for it, as much as politeness allows!

The Dangers Of Snoring

Intimately wrapped with the subject of sleep and yawning is the issue of snoring. Most people laugh at it and think snoring is no more than inconvenient, or perhaps a marker of personal crankiness. In fact snoring is potentially very dangerous.

Approximately 40 percent of adult women, 57 percent of adult men, and 27 percent of children are said to snore.

Snoring is very unhealthy; it ties in closely with sleep apnea, which means unnatural cessation of breathing rhythms for 20 to 30 seconds at a time—Greek *apnea*, meaning "no breath" (obviously, breathing must soon resume, otherwise the person would simply die!)

Sleep apnea is associated with many health problems, including cardiac arrest, hypertension, stroke, obesity, diabetes and a shortened lifespan. Being overweight markedly increases your risk of sleep apnea.

Diagnosis of sleep breathing disorders, such as apnea, is not simple because there can be many different causes. Primary healthcare providers, pulmonologists, neurologists, or other healthcare providers with specialty training in sleep disorders may be involved in making a diagnosis and starting treatment. Several tests are available for evaluating breathing during sleep, including:

- **Polysomnography.** This test records a variety of body functions during sleep, such as brain waves, the oxygen level in your blood, heart rate and breathing, as well as eye and leg movements during the study.

- **Multiple Sleep Latency Test (MSLT).** This test measures the speed of falling asleep. People without sleep problems usually take an average of 10 to 20 minutes to fall asleep. People who fall asleep in less than 5 minutes are likely to need some type of treatment for sleep disorders.

Diagnostic tests usually are done in a sleep center, but new technology may allow some sleep studies to be done in your home, by wearing a device which keeps a record during the night.

Heart Abnormalities

It's not just about generalized ill health but one specific problem is closely tied to sleep apnea and that is an irregular heart beat which is dangerous, though not uniformly fatal by any means.

Obstructive sleep apnea, which involves the partial or complete blockage of airways and is the most common type of sleep-related breathing disorder, is associated with irregular heartbeats; the more severe a patient's sleep-disordered breathing, the greater his risk for arrhythmia.

The study appears in the June 22 issue of the Archives of Internal Medicine.

In 2011, another study went further at the Case Western Reserve University School of Medicine. They studied the link between sleep apnea and atrial fibrillation (AFib), the most commonly diagnosed type of arrhythmia, or irregular heart rhythm.

AFib is characterized by an abnormally rapid heart rate (like a flutter) that can be so fast it doesn't get the blood flowing. The strange thing is that AFib is on the increase, with no known associative factors. It seems highly probable that this increase is due largely to sleep disorders, especially obstructive apnea, says Reena Mehra MD, MS, associate professor of medicine in the Department of Medicine at Case Western Reserve University School of Medicine.

In prior research, Dr. Mehra and her colleagues established a strong association between sleep apnea and AFib, basing their findings on thousands of participants in large scale epidemiologic surveys.

In particular, they found actual physical changes in the hearts of patients with pronounced sleep apnea and AFib tendency.

So it's emerging as more and more important.

The fact is, one billion people suffer from obstructive sleep apnea, according to a 2017 estimate from the WHO. That's one in seven people, so it's no small issue!

In the USA sleep apnea now afflicts at least 25 million adults in the U.S., according to the National Healthy Sleep Awareness Project, published in 2014. Several new studies highlight the destructive nature of obstructive sleep apnea, a chronic disease that increases the risk of high blood pressure, heart disease, Type 2 diabetes, stroke and depression.

[Lancet Respir Med. 2019 Aug; 7(8): 687–698. Published online 2019 Jul 9. doi: 10.1016/S2213-2600(19)30198-5]

What Can Be Done?

Sleep apnea is typically treated with a continuous positive airway pressure (CPAP) machine. This is a device that forces the issue of breathing regularly, by mechanical rhythmical control, via a tube and mask worn in bed. It's very intrusive but patients eventually get used to it and many report sleeping much better and waking refreshed.

It's worth noting that a growing number of dentists insist that a dental prosthesis, designed to maintain a proper airway (breathing pathway) works just as well as a CPAP machine, by pushing the lower jaw forward. This was finally confirmed by a definitive study, published in 2019 in the journal Sleep Disorders.

[Yu Matsumura, Hiroshi Ueda, Toshikazu Nagasaki, Cynthia Concepción Medina, Koji Iwai, Kotaro Tanimoto. Multislice Computed Tomography Assessment of Airway Patency Changes Associated with Mandibular Advancement Appliance Therapy in Supine Patients with Obstructive Sleep Apnea. *Sleep Disorders*, 2019; 2019: 1 DOI: 10.1155/2019/8509820]

As for snoring, there is a whole host of tricks and treatments for sale, from devices that hold open your nostrils, to chinstraps, to mouthpieces, better pillows and herbal tinctures.

How you lie in bed is also crucial: snoring comes about when your tongue drops into the back of your throat and causes a partial obstruction. Thus sleeping on your back is the worst possible sleep position and you are encouraged to sleep on one side or the other.

But for this section we cut to the chase and look at the most effective and totally the most astonishing way to prevent snoring. Ready? It's tape your mouth closed at night!

Say what?

That's right: tape up your mouth! This is a whole new raft of sleep and snoring science, relating to how we breath naturally. There are mouth breathers (not good) and nasal breathers (excellent). Surprisingly, we can force the former into being the latter by preventing mouth breathing altogether.

This comes from a particularly impressive body of work by James Nestor and published in his game-changing book *Breath: The New Science of A Lost Art* (Riverhead Books, 2020).

Nestor examines the history, science, and culture of breathing and its impacts on human health. In the book he investigates the history of how we shifted from the natural state of nasal breathing to chronic mouth breathing and explains research which argues that this shift (due to the increased consumption of processed foods) has led to a rise in snoring, sleep apnea, asthma, autoimmune disease, and allergies. It includes 10 years of research and Nestor's own personal experiences with breathing.

I highly recommend this read. And you can also catch him being interviewed for a podcast, if you are sufficiently motivated, in a 54 min YouTube video here:

LINK: https://www.youtube.com/watch?v=s0EftTC4mYs

Basically, what Nestor found, is that we have lost the art of proper breathing. This seems shocking, because we have been breathing for our whole life. We breathe over 20,000 times a day. How could it be wrong?

Well, look at it this way: we've been eating our whole life. But that doesn't prevent the majority of people eating the wrong things and harming themselves in the process! Breath is just another kind of nutrient. It belongs along with right eating and exercize is as a fundamental of good health.

As with what we eat and what we do, we are not guaranteed anything. We have choices. The trouble is if we breathe wrongly over a period of time, it alters the whole shape of our skulls and that makes the problem anatomically permanent.

As Nestor says, if you don't breathe properly, you are never going to get back to optimum health. Put the other way round, there is a great deal of ill health you can correct simply by changing your breathing habits.

So How Do We Get Back To Proper Breathing?

Nestor recommends taping the mouth, as I said. It's not New Age woo-woo. It's not dangerous! Just do it and forget the "theory". I married into a family of bigtime Olympic snorers and I can speak from some experience. My parents-in-law had to sleep separately, otherwise they would keep each other awake with loud noises!

My lovely wife Vivien tried the taping approach and the benefits were instant. She now no longer snores, sleeps better and is more comfortable on waking than she has been for years! It works, for goodness sake!

Thing is, Nestor isn't a lone voice. It is true that (almost) nobody talks about this. But there have been real scientists studying this effect for decades now.

Nestor has simply been the author to popularize this trick. It's now all over the internet—just ignore what you see there: we don't use duct tape or anything heavy to close off the mouth completely. Just a short length of cloth tape, like 3M micropore. Take a couple of inches maximum and put it VERTICALLY over your mouth, not along the lip line (like a Charlie Chaplin moustache).

Kill the stickiness by handling the tape surface a few times. We are not trying to jam or hold the mouth shut; just send signals to the brain, to remind it to keep your mouth closed through the night. You can always breathe past the tape, so don't be apprehensive.

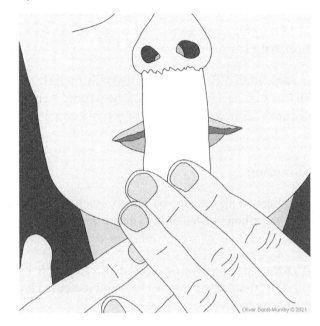

And don't rip it off in the morning! Stick out your tongue and loosen the tape from the inside with saliva.

It's easy!

Finally, if even snoring is a big problem, don't wait for a diagnosis of sleep apnea: fix it!

"You should consult a doctor when snoring is loud, awakens the patient with gasping or choking, or when sleep becomes disrupted and/or you start feeling that your sleep is no longer refreshing, and you are tired, fatigued, blue and/or sleepy during the daytime."

—Alan R. Schwartz, M.D. adjunct professor at the University of Pennsylvania Perelman School of Medicine Professor, and professor at Johns Hopkins University

How To Catch Up On Lost Sleep

Lack of sufficient sleep is called sleep deprivation. It's cumulative and individuals who sleep poorly can be carrying around a backlog of missed sleep that goes back weeks, or even months. *It is highly beneficial to start catching up on your sleep deficit.*

It won't happen with a single early night. If you've had months of restricted sleep, you'll have built up a significant sleep debt and recovery can be expected to take several weeks.

Starting on a weekend, try to add on an extra hour or two of sleep a night. Expect to sleep for upwards of 10 hours a night at first. After a while, the amount of time you sleep will gradually decrease to a normal level.

Here are 7 benefits from sleeping soundly and sufficiently can boost your health, from the UK NHS website:

Boosting Immunity

In times of COVID, this can be specially important! If you seem to catch every cold and flu that's going around, a lack of sleep could be to blame. Prolonged lack of sleep can disrupt your immune system, so you're less able to fend off bugs.

Slimming

Sleeping less may mean you put on weight! Studies have shown that people who sleep less than 7 hours a day tend to gain more weight and have a higher risk of becoming obese than those who get 7 hours of slumber.

It's believed to be because sleep-deprived people have reduced levels of leptin (the chemical that makes you feel full) and increased levels of ghrelin (the hunger-stimulating hormone).

Boosting Mental Wellbeing

Given that a single sleepless night can make you irritable and moody the following day, it's not surprising that chronic sleep debt may lead to long-term mood disorders like depression and anxiety.

When people with anxiety or depression were surveyed to calculate their sleeping habits, it turned out that most of them slept for less than 6 hours a night.

Studies using different methods and populations estimate that 65% to 90% of adult patients with major depression, and about 90% of children with this disorder, experience some kind of sleep problem. Most patients with depression have insomnia, but about one in five suffer also from obstructive sleep apnea.

Sleep Prevents Diabetes

Studies have suggested that people who usually sleep less than 5 hours a night have an increased risk of developing diabetes.

It seems that missing out on deep sleep may lead to type 2 diabetes by changing the way the body processes glucose, which the body uses for energy.

Sleep Increases Sex Drive

Yes to this one! Men and women who don't get enough quality sleep have lower libidos and less of an interest in sex, research suggests.

Men who suffer from sleep apnoea – a disorder in which breathing difficulties lead to interrupted sleep – also tend to have lower testosterone levels, which can in turn lower libido.

Sleep Wards Off Heart Disease

Long-standing sleep deprivation seems to be associated with increased heart rate, an increase in blood pressure and higher levels of certain chemicals linked with inflammation, which may put extra strain on your heart.

Sleep Increases Fertility

A pleasant shock and great news with couples struggling with infertility!

Difficulty conceiving a baby has been claimed as one of the effects of sleep deprivation, in both men and women. Apparently, regular sleep disruptions can cause trouble conceiving by reducing the secretion of reproductive hormones.

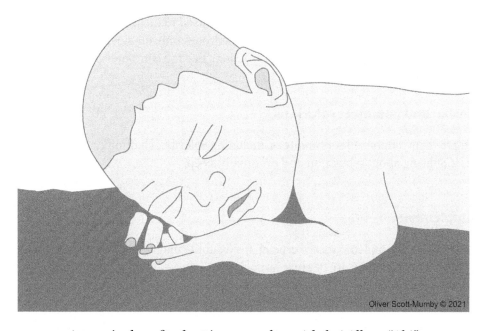

A surprise benefit of getting more sleep. A baby! All say "Ah!"

Part 2. Getting To Sleep

OK, enough preliminaries. Let's get down to it... How do we actually approach getting adequate healthful sleep? Best solution, of course, is a clear mind and a happy heart. You are at peace with the world. Nothing could rock your calm and gentle nature. All is good. Falling asleep is the most natural thing in...

BANG! It's just not like that any more. The world is hostile, violent, threatening, confusing and scary. What to do? Even sane and clever people are confused, scared, feeling insecure.

The threat to sleep is now wrapped up with the threat to social order, global warming, terrorist threats, pandemics (real or otherwise) and the remote possibility (magnified by the media to an near certainty) of an asteroid impact.

How can anyone go to bed and sleep in peace, I ask you?

Actions to take in the case of troublesome insomnia come in several categories:

1. Preparation

Preparing the environment, removing distractions and setting the right conditions for good sleep. Good "sleep hygiene" is the term often used to include tips like maintaining a regular sleep-and-wake schedule, using the bedroom only for sleeping or sex, and keeping the bedroom dark and free of distractions like the computer or television.

2. Herbal and botanical solutions

There are many famous plants and teas, including valerian, chamomile and lemon balm, that bring about relaxation and eventually sleep.

3. Supplements

Some nutritional supplements are crucial, for example magnesium, known as "nature's tranquillizer". B vitamins are of great importance to nerve function and deficiency of any of the B vitamins can lead to restlessness, anxiety, tension and the jitters. Not good for sleep!

4. Metabolic substances

There is a whole raft of substances our bodies need which affect sleep. Without adequate supply, we have trouble getting off and remaining asleep. Our brain needs adequate inositol, for example, and a related substance called GABA (gamma aminobutyric acid). These substances are generally classified as neuro-transmitters or signaling molecules and gain more and more importance, as we learn more about neurological functioning.

5. Homeopathic Remedies

Homeopathy is one of the most wonderful and advanced healing modalities ever created. It enjoys a huge reputation worldwide. Hundreds of millions of people swear by it in India, for example, because it is effective and costs next to nothing (pennies on the dollar).

There are several good homeopathic sleeping remedies shared here, which you may experiment with. Try to match the OTHER symptoms to the remedy. There is no remedy that will work the same for everyone, but hey... isn't that nature? We are all different.

6. Hormonal balancing

Melatonin is the best-known sleep substance. It truly is a sleep hormone. But it's not quite as simple as that. If an individual's other hormones are out of balance, he (or usually a she) will have difficulty coping in life... and that includes the ability to sleep. If you are in biochemical turmoil, that's not good for your chances of sound sleep.

The book does not go into details of matters such as PMS, PMDD (pre-menstrual dysphoric disorder) and the menopause, because they really are beyond self-help medication. But these conditions truly impact sleeping and you will need to get help if your inability to sleep properly stems from these and similar hormonal disorders.

7. Mechanical and electronic aids

I have already mentioned the in then 19th century machine. These may have a part to play. But I get much more excited about electronic devices and their ability to favorably alter brain function.

That's particularly true of brain entrainment leading to slower brain wave states, such as alpha and theta relaxation. More of that later.

8. Energy work

What about acupuncture? Why not? It works in general. In fact some limited science does demonstrate that it has a place. The results suggest that insomnia patients may experience significant improvement in symptoms after more than three weeks of acupuncture treatment. At core, acupuncture is about adjusting Ch'i energy around the body. There are other ways to do this.

9. Psychological and inner deep work

Of course our mental and biological state is influenced by how we feel in life, feel about life, and the thoughts, ideas, beliefs, patterns and reactive patterns we experience.

If you lie awake tossing and turning half the night, because you are stressed, fearful, depressed or anxious, that will ruin your quality of sleep. So this is something we have to talk about, for this to be a comprehensive book.

At the end of the day, life is an experience and how we respond to circumstances we meet is really at the core of what we are pleased to call "the quality of life." What we get back depends on what we put in... and that can always be changed!

10. The Desperation Remedy... works every time!

Step 1. Prepare For Sleep

Most people omit a "wind down" step before they go to bed. This is a serious mistake.

You need to slow down or stop mental stimulation at least one hour before retiring. That means no TV, no texting, no WhatsApp calls, no online games, no sugary drinks, no alcohol, and of course NO CAFFEINE! Don't forget: nicotine is a strong stimulant, which speeds heart rate and thinking.

Also turn OFF the electronic devices, such as computers, tablets, TV and smartphones. Better still, get rid of them out of your sleeping space. WIFI and EMF radiation can reach you even if you are not actually talking with a friend.

A far better idea than "entertainment" would be a warm shower or tub soak before you go to bed! Maybe a massage, if you have a spouse or loving friend who will administer it. Adding lavender or other essential oils may bring even more benefit, though so-called "essential oil therapy" is beyond this book (the word essential comes from "essences", meaning the scented oils).

Part of the preparation process is to take control of your physical environment. We want SILENCE. If that's not achievable, you must use earplugs to dampen the ambient noise.

Light is stressful, especially blue light. Blue light damages your eyes and that is now a recognized hazard of using computers: computer monitors emit bluish light, unless accompanied by a software app, such as f.lux, which turns your screen to yellow at a set point in the evening (back to white next morning).

For optimum sleep we need the bedroom as dark as possible. Don't worry about fancy fabrics, designer drapes and screens: we want a black out, if possible. Who cares how it looks?

If you can't achieve reasonable darkness, get a sleep mask. They are quite comfortable and you'll soon get used to wearing one.

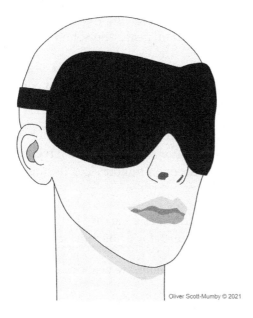

Oliver Scott-Mumby © 2021

Sleep mask for complete blackout

2. Herbal and Botanical Solutions

Sleep remedies are things you do, or take, to help put you to sleep and (preferably) keep you asleep for many hours—not the same thing, note.

A good place to start is with amino acid L-Theanine. It's a herbal nutrient present in black tea, from the Camelia bush, which may explain why tea has such a calming effect on the whole. But it's better to buy the remedy from the health foods store: the dose is guaranteed and can be controlled. Take 100 mg at first, if that's not enough, try 200 mg. If that doesn't work, try something else.

Important note: L-Theanine will knock you out but does not hold you in sleep. Hence a quiet and darkened ambience is important. You don't want waking up again after just 2 – 3 hours sleep!

California Poppy

Other names: Eschscholzia, Meconopsis, Amapola de California, Pavot d'Amérique, Pavot d'Or, Pavot de Californie, Yellow Poppy)

California poppy, although now found in gardens all over the world, is indigenous to California and has been used by Native Americans as a sedative, hypnotic, and analgesic. It remains widely popular among herbal practitioners today as a powerful treatment for sleep disorders, especially overexcitement and sleeplessness, and also as an antispasmodic when there is muscular tension, restlessness, and pain.

It was even used by medical practitioners and sold by Park-Davis as an excellent alternative to morphine without its side effects (California poppy is not addictive and does not cause the adverse effects associated with opiates).

Animal studies have demonstrated the binding of alkaloids in California poppy to GABA receptors. It has an affinity for the benzodiazepine (valium, etc.) receptor. Eschshcolzia should be considered when there is the need to promote sleep during periods of serious stress.

It can be taken as a tea, but is often prescribed as a sedative in tincture form to be taken in small repeated doses every 15 to 30 minutes for 2 hours prior to attempting to sleep.

[https://www.sciencedirect.com/topics/biochemistry-genetics-and-molecular-biology/eschscholzia]

Chamomile

Try Chamomile tea. Chamomile (*Matricaria camomilla*) is a common flowering plant that is indigenous to various parts of central and southern Europe. The dried leaves and flowers are commonly packaged as a tea and can be purchased over the counter in both bagged and loose form.

Unlike some herbal sleep remedies, chamomile does not have to be used on a regular basis to be effective as a treatment for insomnia. It can be used on the spot to provide quick relief for sleeplessness and anxiety.

Chamomile tea is most effective when sipped a half an hour to forty-five minutes before going to bed. It has been found that chamomile can be especially helpful in relieving the symptoms of mild insomnia (a.k.a. transient insomnia).

Chrysin, a flavonoid component of Chamomile, is the chemical attributed to Chamomile's ability to relieve anxiety and promote sleep. Chrysin can also be found in Passionflower (*Passiflora incarnatus*), another plant that has been found to be effective in the treatment of insomnia and anxiety.

Other teas with restful possibilities include Lemon balm, Melissa and tilleul (aka. lime or linden). You can also get combinations of different relaxing teas. Try a bunch and choose the one that has the best results for you.

3. Nutritional Supplements

Magnesium is one of nature's wonder healing substances. It is vital for healthy nerve functioning and is crucial for about 500 different biochemical enzyme transformation pathways. Not surprisingly, therefore, a lack of magnesium can lead to a great diversity of symptoms.

Many of magnesium's important functions are connected with the nervous system. Lack of magnesium causes a state of over excitability, with twitching, tremors, anxiety, hyperactivity, cramps, convulsions and insomnia. Because it counters such symptoms, magnesium has been christened 'Nature's tranquillizer'.

Paradoxically, a lack of magnesium is a major factor in fatigue (a depressed, rather than excited state). This is almost certainly because magnesium is essential for the phase I detoxification pathway. Lack of magnesium can lead to an increase in unwanted metabolites such as chloral hydrate ('Mickey Finn'), giving rise to a 'spacey' and tired feeling.

A lack of magnesium can also lead to raised blood-pressure and heart abnormalities. PMS seems to benefit greatly from magnesium supplementation, probably because it is needed in metabolizing omega-3 essential fatty acids, which are famously anti-inflammatory and therefore anti-pain.

Magnesium makes a great analgesic and if pain keeps you awake at night, especially musculo-skeletal pain (backache, etc.), magnesium is worth a try.

Despite its importance, there is no known test to substantiate how much magnesium is that the average diet provides only about 40 per cent of even the Recommended Daily Allowance (RDA)! Soils are depleted of magnesium due to acid rain; food processing removes a great deal of magnesium and high phosphates in the diet interfere with its absorption (colas and other fizzy drinks are high in phosphates).

Those especially at risk are alcohol drinkers, individuals with inflammatory gut disease, whether due to infection or allergies, and joggers and health buffs, who sweat a great deal. Overdoing it in the gym, without supplementing magnesium, may not be so healthy.

Dose: 200 to 800 mg daily. Care may be needed in supplementations as it can lead to diarrhea and a worsening in magnesium status, due to a loss of electrolytes from the colon.

Intravenous Magnesium

If the patient's status warrants it, intravenous administration of magnesium may be recommended by a physician. One gram is administered in a 2-ml syringe, slowly into a vein in the arm.

It causes a wonderful warm, relaxing "glow" (literally!), probably due to peripheral vasodilatation, leading to increased blood flow in the skin.

I remember in the 1980s and 90s my circle of clinical ecology friends, at gatherings and meetings, injecting each other with magnesium for back pain. It worked, so why not?

Magnesium had a short vogue as treatment for acute cardiac conditions, where arrhythmia (irregular beat) was a hazard. It wasn't long before Big Pharma had this cheap and unpatentable substitute for their expensive drugs trashed by fake science and it has slipped out of fashion.

Whenever you want to think "calming" think "magnesium?"

Vitamin C

By now my readers will know I think of vitamin C as the greatest healer on earth. It's also important for cardiovascular health, and necessary for the body to make collagen, which is critical for healthy bones, teeth, and skin.

But vitamin C may also extend and improve sleep.

A 2013 study by scientists at the University of Pennsylvania found that short sleepers—people who slept less than 6 hours a night—consumed less vitamin C than people who consumed more of the vitamin. Lower levels of vitamin C, as measured in the blood, were also linked to more nightly sleep disturbance and a greater risk for sleep disorders.

On its own and in combination with other antioxidants, vitamin C has been shown to improve the symptoms of obstructive sleep apnea. A 2009 study showed that a combination of vitamin C (100 mg) and vitamin E (400 IU) taken twice daily reduced episodes of apnea. This C and E combination also improved sleep quality and decreased daytime sleepiness.

I think we need far more than 100 mg of vitamin C a day. Goats and other animals make their own: around 12 grams a day (12,000 mg!) My special well-tolerated formula is design to avoid bowel irritation (abdominal pain and diarrhea)—you can find it at www.DrKeithsOwn.com

B Vitamins

Inositol is part of the B complex but dealt with in the next section.

B complex is a battery of essential nutrients, including thiamine (B1), riboflavin (B2), niacin (B3), pyridoxine (B6), folic acid and others. The B's are important building blocks and provide essential support for your immune system, skin and central nervous system, the latter of which monitors many of the chemical processes involved with mood and sleep.

When your body is deficient in any of the major B vitamins (a common finding) early symptoms could include depression and insomnia. Some people have reported that insomnia symptoms have diminished noticeably once they begin a regular routine of taking B-complex vitamins, a supplement that packages all the B's together.

B6 is important. A lack has been linked to symptoms of insomnia and depression. Vitamin B6 aids in the production of the hormones serotonin and melatonin, both of which are important to sound, restful sleep, and also to mood.

You can find B6 in milk, eggs, cheese, fish, bananas, carrots, spinach, potatoes, and whole grains.

Vitamin B12 is important for brain function, supporting cardiovascular health including red blood cell formation, and in supporting DNA activity. Here's what we know about its effects on sleep.

Several studies have demonstrated that this vitamin is involved in regulating sleep-wake cycles by helping to keep circadian rhythms in sync. Some studies show a connection between low vitamin B12 and insomnia, while other studies show higher levels of vitamin B12 are linked to sleep disruption and shorter sleep times.

Higher levels of vitamin B12 have been equated with a lower risk of depression. People who are depressed tend to sleep badly, so they may be directly connected.

[SOURCE: Psychology Today: https://www.psychologytoday.com/us/blog/sleep-new-zzz/201905/5-ways-vitamin-deficiencies-can-impact-your-sleep]

So, we want adequate, not excess. The best way to maintain your B12 levels if you are over 50 is to have regular injections of hydroxycobalamin: 1,000 mcg (1 mg) monthly is good.

B12 is found in Vitamin B12 is found in animal protein dietary sources, including dairy, eggs, meat, fish, and shellfish.

Magnesium-Melatonin-B Complex Mixture

I found an interesting 2019 study, which compared a mix of magnesium, melatonin and B complex for insomnia. The results were not outstanding but definitely significant, turning moderate insomnia into "mild" insomnia, according to ratings on the Athens insomnia scale: 15 points, down to 10 points. That's a drop of around 30%!

That could make the difference between enough sleep and not enough sleep, for some individuals. In the words of the researchers, "Magnesium-melatonin-B complex supplementation has a beneficial effect in the treatment of insomnia regardless of cause."

[Open Access Maced J Med Sci. 2019 Sep 30; 7(18): 3101–3105. Published online 2019 Aug 30]

Vitamin D

For a whole host of reasons, you cannot afford to be deficient in vitamin D. It's vital for the full functioning of the immune system and that means protection against bacteria, viruses AND cancer.

Thing is, a deficiency in vitamin D is linked to lessened sleep quality and shorter sleep time (time spent asleep), especially in those over 50. But there is more to it than that. Vitamin D is a very powerful vitamin which impacts some 800 genes. Deficiency of it may prevent the working of two genes responsible for our circadian clocks—which control our 24-hour circadian rhythm. Our circadian rhythm tells us when to go to sleep and when to wake up. It's not just choice: our bodies really won't wake up properly until cortisol levels rise for the day.

The only way to be sure you have adequate blood levels is lab testing. You doctor should know what's what but, if he or she does not, you can run the show and aim for levels of 25-hydroxy vitamin D of at least 40 – 50 nanograms/milliliter to 50 ng/mL. Ignore stupid orthodox advice which consider 20 nanograms to be adequate. Not even close!

4. Metabolic substances

GABA

You could consider 500 – 1,000 mg of GABA (gamma-aminobutyric acid), a nerve relaxant. GABA has been dubbed the Valium of the natural world but don't be fooled by marketing hoaxes. However, it does bring relaxation and induces sleep.

A 2018 study published in the journal *Molecules* suggests that breathing in the scent of jasmine (a substance frequently used in aromatherapy) may help enhance the effects of GABA. It could be something to try this oil over a candle in your bedroom [Wang ZJ, Heinbockel T. Essential oils and their constituents targeting the GABAergic system and sodium channels as treatment of neurological diseases. *Molecules*. 2018;23(5):1061. doi:10.3390/molecules23051061

Inositol

Inositol (aka. myo-inositol) is intimately related to GABA and uses the same receptors. It is found naturally in foods such as fruits, beans, grains and nuts.

Inositol helps promote a feeling of calmness and peacefulness, which are the main factors in helping someone get a good night of sleep. Inositol can help improve communication throughout the brain, which is done by releasing neurotransmitters like serotonin.

Sleep requires good serotonin levels in the body. If you have depleted serotonin levels, you will often feel like your mind cannot shut down at night, which triggers endless thoughts that can be similar to someone who is overly compulsive. The better your serotonin levels are, the less likely you will have these types of endless thoughts when your head hits the pillow, and a more restful sleep will occur

Inositol works best when it's taken regularly! The typical dose ranges anywhere from 500 mg to 2000 mg and it should be taken it at night a few hours before you go to bed. You need to take it consistently and the benefits will come!

5. Homeopathic Solutions

Surprisingly, even holistic practitioners remain hostile to homeopathy, on the grounds, "It can't possibly work, therefore it is useless or a fraud."

Be assured it is highly effective and valuable, subject to choosing the right remedy for the right person (this is not like orthodox pharmacy, where everyone is affected similarly). For example, a woman who could not sleep because she was recently bereaved would not qualify for the same remedy as a woman who could not sleep because of fear, anxiety and panic attacks.

The huge benefit of homeopathy is its extremely high safety margin since, as critics love to point out, some "potencies" (dilutions) are so great that no possible chemical substance can be present. But that's not to say that the active principle is not still present. It is—and that's the whole point! It's just not "stuff" (active molecules); it's energy and information!

The key principle of homeopathy is that "Like cures like". So a remedy that causes sore throat would be used to treat a sore throat (subject to critical dilutions). Caffeine, which causes restlessness and jitters instead of sleep, could be used to cure wakefulness; again, subject to critical dilutions.

ALL VERY CONTROVERSIAL. But remember, homeopathy is over 2 centuries old in proving itself. Current drug pharmacy practice barely 50 years and has NOT proven itself very effective.

Astonishingly, the KaiserPermanente website lists a whole range of homeopathic sleep remedies! (https://wa.kaiserpermanente.org/kbase/topic.jhtml?docId=hn-2258008)

These are just a few of my choices...

Coffea cruda

Made from unroasted coffee beans, the homeopathic remedy coffea cruda claims to have the exact opposite effect as a cup of joe: it unwinds the mind instead of revving it up, and is most often used to combat sleeplessness and racing thoughts in children and adults with ADHD.

Avena Sativa

Provides relief from fatigue and exhaustion and helps in restoring energy levels. it corrects sleeping disorders and promotes better sleep.

Nux vomica

This remedy relieves irritability, sleeplessness at 3 a.m., and digestive troubles associated with overindulgence in food, tobacco or alcohol.

Silicea (also called Silica)

This is a useful remedy for nervous people with low stamina who get too tired, then have insomnia. The person often goes to sleep at first, but awakens suddenly with a hot or surging feeling in the head—and finds it hard to fall asleep again. People who need this remedy usually have anxious dreams, and some (especially children) sleepwalk frequently.

Sulphur

This remedy may be helpful if insomnia comes from itching—or an increasing feeling of heat in bed, especially in the feet. The person is irritable and anxious, and often feels hot and wants to throw the covers off. Lying awake between two and five a.m. is typical. Insomnia that develops because of a lack of exercise may also be helped with *Sulphur*.

Aconitum napellus (monk's hood or wolfsbane)

This remedy, from the buttercup family, can be helpful if a person panics with insomnia. Fear and agitation come on suddenly when the person is drifting off to sleep, or may even wake a sleeping person up.

Arnica montana

This remedy relieves pain and restless sleep from muscle overexertion.

Rhus Tox

This is also good for tired, aching muscles and is useful for sleeplessness due to overdoing things.

Arsenicum album

People who need this remedy are often anxious and compulsive about small details, and have trouble sleeping if they feel that everything is not in place. They are often deeply weary and exhausted, yet feel restless physically and mentally. Sleep, when it arrives, can be anxious and disturbed, with dreams full of fear and insecurity.

Calcarea phosphorica

This remedy is often helpful to children with growing pains, and also to adults who have aching in the joints and bones, or neck and shoulder tension that make it hard to fall asleep. The person who needs this remedy lies awake for many hours, feeling upset and irritable—then has trouble waking in the morning, feeling deeply tired and weak.

Cocculus

This remedy is often helpful to those who feel "too tired to sleep" after long-term sleep loss—from getting up with an infant, taking care of someone who is ill, a disruptive work schedule, travel and jet lag, or chronic worry and insomnia. The person may feel weak and dizzy, with trouble thinking, and may be sleepy, irritable, or tearful.

Ignatia

If insomnia is caused by emotional upset (grief or loss, a disappointment in love, a shock, or even an argument) this remedy may be helpful. The person is sensitive and nervous, and may often sigh and yawn in the daytime, but find it hard to relax at night. As the person tries to fall asleep, the arms and legs may twitch or itch. If sleep arrives, it is usually light, with jerking of the legs and arms, or long and troubling nightmares.

Lycopodium

People who need this remedy often have no memory of dreams and often doubt that they have slept at all. Insomnia may set in primarily because of worry: lack of confidence can make them doubt their own abilities, although they are usually very capable. Ravenous hunger in the night that wakes a person up is another indication for *Lycopodium*.

But don't forget middle of the night is a classic time for low blood sugar too.

Zincum metallicum

People who need this remedy often have insomnia from mental activity. They can get wound up from overwork—or be naturally inclined toward nervousness and just have trouble relaxing. Their legs and arms often feel extremely restless, and lying still in bed may be impossible. Even during the daytime, a person who needs this remedy may feel a constant need to move the muscles.

6. Hormonal Balancing

Melatonin

Everyone knows melatonin. It is secreted by the pineal gland and is a powerful anti-oxidant, as well as a sleep hormone. It can leave you groggy, so don't take too much; 3 mg is about right for an adult. If you find yourself waking too soon, try the sustained-release form (SR). It delivers melatonin slowly over several hours to maintain blood levels for a longer period of time.

Better is to take a self-concocted sleep formula, as follows:

- 3 mgs melatonin
- 5,000 IU of vitamin D
- 50 – 100 mg of 5-hydroxytryptophan (5HT)
- 400 mg of magnesium citrate

This suggestion comes from my good friend Graham Simpson MD and he swears by it.

Vitex Agnus Castus

The herb *Vitex agnus castus* (chaste tree, chaste berry) may help insomnia and sleep disturbances associated with menstrual periods and menopause. In one study, women were treated with a combination of agnus castus and magnolia extracts combined with soy isoflavones and lactobacilli. This treatment was found to be safe and effective over a one-year period. [De Franciscis P, Grauso F, Luisi A, Schettino MT, Torella M, Colacurci N. Adding agnus castus and magnolia to soy isoflavones relieves sleep disturbances besides postmenopausal vasomotor symptoms--long term safety and effectiveness. *Nutrients.* 2017;9(2). doi:10.3390/nu9020129]

However, chaste-berry should not be used by anyone on birth control pills, hormone replacement therapy, or dopamine-related medications, according to the National Center for Complementary and Integrative Health. [National Center for Complementary and Integrative Health. Chasteberry. U.S. Department of Health and Human Services. Updated September 2016. nccih.nih.gov]

Thyroid Gland

An overactive of underactive thyroid gland can cause sleep problems. Underactive thyroid (hypothyroidism) causes weight gain and is known to increase the risk of snoring, obesity, obstructive sleep breathing disorders and sleep apnea.

An overactive thyroid (hyperthyroidism) leads to excess energy, agitation, anxiety, restlessness and, of course, insomnia.

[Lencu C, Alexescu T, Petrulea M, Lencu M. Respiratory manifestations in endocrine diseases. Clujul Med. 2016;89(4):459-463. doi:10.15386/cjmed-671]

Proper diagnosis and correction of thyroid dysfunction is beyond the scope of this book. But since I already know in advance that your doctor or specialist will make a mess of fixing it (they nearly always do!), let me tell you to get real and valuable information from my friend Janie Bowthorpe, who runs a terrific self-help website for thyroid sufferers called: StopTheThyroidMadness.com

PMS, PMDD, Adrenal Insufficiency

There are some other pretty serious hormonal-based conditions. Once again, you will probably need help to get it fixed.

Good luck with that!

7. Electronic Sleep Aid Devices

Wearable meditation technology, so called

Alpha brain entrainment devices are available in the market and online. This is now usually grouped all together as "wearable meditation technology", for example the Muse, Flowtime and Alpha Stim.

But I'd like to share with you, in some detail, what I consider the best of all electronic devices for inducing calm, deep and lasting sleep. It's called the BrainTap.

This is brain entrainment at its best. It has four modalities which will put you to sleep, restfully and composed, by reducing your brainwave frequency. There are binaural beats, flickering lights (so-called photic driving), relaxing peaceful music, and my voice, droning on gently, taking you on inspiring "creative mind walks"—all together on the same restful track!

Some people say they can't even get to the end of my tracks, because they are already asleep!

Here are some notes to help you understand what's different. I call it:

Electronic Zen

Everyone knows that meditation is soothing and calming, you relax, your blood pressure comes down and you live longer (well, almost everyone knows).

I used to do it when I was at med school. I had a big passion for all things Japanese, especially Zen Buddhism. I wrote a special form of poetry called *Haiku* and I won a round-the-world trip for one I wrote in 1967. I worked it out as several hundred dollars per syllable prize money!

The trouble is, it takes many years to get good at meditation. Some say 30 years.

How about if we could get all the health benefits of meditation in less than 10 minutes? Sounds good?

This is where Western energy medicine comes into its own. I've been promoting the idea that our Western version of energy medicine won't be some wishy washy make over of Chinese or Indian models (which are just as riddled with dogma as Western science).

In the West we have something better to offer: electronic and technical brilliance. We are already w-a-y past anything the Chinese could do with acupuncture. That's old-fashioned, crude and rather brutal, actually, shoving needles into people. Ugh!

It's much smarter to project red laser light into the acupuncture points and you can even have the light carry the electronic "signature" of remedies. I covered all this in my earth-shaking book *Medicine Beyond* [www.MedicineBeyond.com].

Electronic Meditation

Let's get back to electronic gadgets and their ability to modulate biological parameters and so influence health.

You will have heard of binaural beats and their ability to entrain brain frequencies. Done well, it can take a person from highly buzzed "*beta waves*", to soothing, calm, relaxed *alpha* or even *theta* brain states.

Binaural beat technology has been around since the 1970s. The first big step came with a ground-breaking paper entitled "Auditory Beats in the Brain" by Dr. Gerald Oster of Mt. Sinai Medical Center, published in the October 1973 issue of *Scientific American*. [Oster, Gerald. (1973). Auditory beats in the brain. Scientific American, 229, 94-102]

Oster introduced the term binaural beats, which occurred in the brain when sounds of different frequencies were presented separately to each ear.

A "beat" is the difference between those two frequencies. Thus if one ear gets 440 cycles per second and the other ear get 444 cycles per second, the resulting beat (the difference between the two) is 4 beats per second.

What happens is that the entire brain then resonates at 4 cycles per second. That just happens to be theta brainwave frequency (4- 7 cycles per second) and is characteristic of deeply relaxed, trance-like states.

Good, huh?

Photic Driving

But it gets better; far better. These days we can add flickering lights, which seem to drive the brain even more powerfully than just binaural beats, particularly in the alpha and theta frequencies. This effect was discovered in the 1940s by researcher Gray Walter.

Add slow Baroque music, which has scientifically-proven health enhancements and we get a terrific healing, relaxing technology.

All that needs adding is my sweet, gentle voice (ahem!), guiding you on sensual and exciting mental imagery explorations, such as visiting the Isle of Avalon, Atlantis, galaxies and deep space, talking to our Sun, and we have a stunning combination that makes relaxing mental states, including sleep, not just easy but irresistible! You practically can't fight it! You'll be down in deep alpha or theta before you know it.

A Bit Of Theory

Robert Monroe of the Monroe Institute of Applied Sciences investigated binaural beats, which he famously used to generate "out of body" experiences in himself and others.

In thousands of experiments, using an EEG machine to monitor subject's electrical brain wave patterns, Monroe verified that he could indeed entrain brain wave patterns using binaural beats. Most importantly, he showed that the response did not only happen in the area of the brain responsible for hearing, or only in one hemisphere or the other, but the entire brain responded in harmony, the wave forms of both hemispheres becoming identical in frequency, amplitude, phase, and coherence.

Many researchers have since verified this phenomenon. Language and speech pathologist Dr. Suzanne Evans Morris, Ph.D., says "Research supports the theory that different frequencies presented to each ear through stereo headphones...create a difference tone (or binaural beat) as the brain puts together the two tones it actually hears. Through EEG monitoring the difference tone is identified by a change in the electrical pattern produced by the brain.

Many scientists working in the field have now confirmed, unequivocally, through brain-wave EEG monitoring, that binaural beats have a powerful health and bioregulatory effect.

What Can It Do For YOU?

Almost anything you want!

Over and over this new technology has been scientifically demonstrated to change physiology and our mental landscape. You can use it in whatever direction you wish:

- Weight loss
- Stress busting
- Giving up addictions
- Improved sexual prowess
- More reactivity
- Better behavior patterns
- Improved moods
- Lowering blood pressure
- Learning a language
- Busting out of study failures.
- Kids subjected to this technology can shed ADD and ADHD.
- Pain relief without drugs
- Coping with cancer and other stressful diseases
- And... of course, improved sleep!

Sleep Induction

Dr. Arthur Hastings, PhD., in a paper entitled "Tests of the Sleep Induction Technique" described the effects of subjects listening to a cassette tape specially engineered to slow the brain wave patterns from a normal waking "beta" brain wave pattern to a slower alpha pattern, then to a still slower theta pattern (the brain wave pattern of dreaming sleep), and finally to a delta pattern, the slowest of all, the brain-wave pattern of dreamless sleep.

Hastings says: We were able to test the effects of the sleep tape on brain waves with an EEG machine through the courtesy of the researchers at the Langely-Porter Neuropsychiatric Institute, part of the University of California Medical School in San Francisco. Dr Joe Kaniya, Director of the Psychophysiology of Consciousness Laboratory, monitored the brain-wave frequencies of one subject as he listened to the sleep tape.

The chart recording showed a typical sleep onset pattern: initial alpha waves, then a slowing of the brain waves with sleep spindles, and finally a pattern of stage 2 and 3 sleep brain waves in the low theta range...the patterns in the various stages demonstrated that the tape was influencing the subject's state. [Hastings, Arthur. Tests of the sleep induction technique. Also a privately published manuscript, 1975]

Of course these days audio is much simpler, using MP3 files, instead of casette tapes, which are easily damaged.

Relaxation Response

The production of alpha and theta patterns in the brain correlates well with Harvard mind-body medicine pioneer Herbert Benson's "Relaxation Response", which is the exact opposite of the "fight or flight response." The fight or flight adrenalin response takes blood flow away from the brain and toward the periphery of the body, increases heart rate, blood pressure and breathing, etc. In this state, learning abilities, as well as other mental functions including problem solving and reasoning ability, are markedly inhibited.

[Benson, Herbert. The Relaxation Response. New York: Morrow, 1975]

The ability to reconcile and resolve disputes is also impaired. Quarrelsome? Not good!

The relaxation response, on the other hand, mobilizes us for inward activity by reducing heart rate and blood pressure, relaxing muscles, and increasing the percentage of oxygen flow to the brain. As one might expect, the fight or flight response is accompanied by low amplitude, high frequency beta brain wave patterns in the brain, while the relaxation response so beneficial to learning and problem solving is accompanied by high amplitude, low frequency alpha and theta rhythms.

Good for the mind; good for the soul.

The Brain Tap Device

In this day and age, we all need one of these devices. It's the perfect, soothing answer to modern stressful living.

The best device I know is called the BrainTap and its developer, Dr. Patrick Porter, has helped to integrate my spoken mind journeys into his system. Among them: A Visit To Avalon, Journey To Atlantis, Tour of The Universe, Our Sun Meditation, Love, Gratitude, Forgiveness and "white light" (for pain).

Many people complain that, despite having these tracks included, they can never get to the end of one. They always fall asleep first!

Most importantly, there is a dedicated "sleep track" that's sure to put you to sleep, with its hidden brain induction, and my metaphors for getting to sleep (NOT including counting sheep, ahem!)

My additional tracks come FREE with your purchase of the device, in addition to the many factory-installed tracks. There is a small monthly fee for membership (not obligatory) and you can choose among thousands of other tracks. Just follow your fancy!

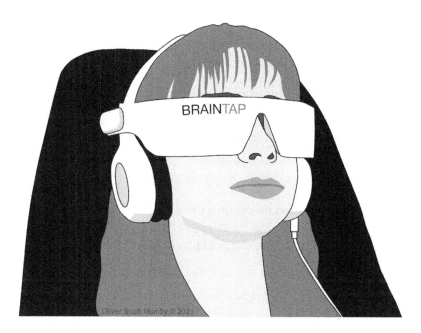

There is a special smartphone app to accompany the BrainTap headset and ganz frames (goggles) set up. It's a delightful experience, comfortable to use and very easy.

Get yourself a BrainTap device here:

alternative-doctor.com/braintap

The Avazzia Device

Good as the BrainTap is, there may be something better. I am thinking of a device with almost identical sleep driving properties—but which can do other things besides brain entrainment, meaning that if you invest in one of these you'll be able to do so MUCH more health-wise than just sleep better.

You will be able to solve pain, heal wounds, terminate infections rapidly, adjust posture, even use it as a defibrillator, and discover a whole host of other benefits that make this device one of the finest health and healing tools in the world. It's a property known as microcurrent therapy (sometimes bioelectric medicine) and is clearly the future.

I'm talking about the Avazzia family of products and I have described the major of these tools as "a hospital in your hand". That's how powerful it is.

It flips the switch on inflammation. Inflammation is what lies behind all pain and disease states. A swift inflammatory response is nature's own healing method. But when the switch gets stuck in the "ON" position, we call that chronic inflammation and it ages you faster than any other process.

In fact I introduced it to the world (originally) as the Russian SCENAR, for which I coined the term "Star Trek Medicine" (*Virtual Medicine*, Thorson's Harper Collins, London, 1999). That was because it seemed to me we were on the brink of a new era in which electronic devices would resemble the small hand-held device used by "Bones" (Leonard McCoy) in the original Star Trek series.

With it, the doctor just clicked a button and the patient could grow a new hand (well, almost!)

Science fiction aside, what a microcurrent therapy device can do is treat inflammation and arthritis, Alzheimer's, heart disease, diabetes, colitis, asthma, autoimmune disease and even cancer, are all chronic inflammatory processes.

To be "inflamed" (on fire) is a good descriptive word for the process that goes on in our bodies. Poor sleep is just one of the inevitable side-effects of generalized inflammation. But poor sleep also CAUSES inflammation; what you Americans call a double-whammy! We need to quench the flames.

So, every home should have one of these devices in the medicine cabinet. It's much more useful than pills and salves.

Moreover, brain entrainment settings are available at the touch of a button, switching to alpha (gentle relaxation), theta (trance, dreaming and meditation) and delta (deep sleep and unconsciousness). This is in addition to pain and healing.

In addition there is a new Gamma frequency settings to help with amazing things like Alzheimer's, PTSD, Anxiety, ADD, ADHD and drug resistant depression (need I say there is science to back all these possibilities).

And if that's not enough: dosing for unrelenting chronic pain, regional pain syndrome, electrical balance, increase in blood flow, fluid reduction in joints and repetitive stress injuries (RSI).

Wow! That's pretty amazing in so small a device and SO MUCH MORE than was possible before. Watch a webinar I hosted about this equipment here: https://vimeo.com/384042638

Today's Big Joke

It seems that bioelectrical healing (their preferred term) has gone mainstream!

One is reminded more than ever of the old adage, that discovery goes through four stages:

1. It's quackery and nonsense

2. There might be something in it

3. There might be something in it but where's the proof?

4. We knew that all along!

Stage 2 (anecdotal evidence, so-called), is where we are supposed to be at. But how long does anecdotal remain a valid accusation? If orthodoxy simply ignores the pioneering work of Robert Becker, Andrew Marino and Joe Spadaro and the many other published authors in this field, does that mean evidence is still anecdotal? How is a large body of peer-reviewed and published research on micro-currents and voltages in healing in bone and other tissues considered "anecdotal"?

The Medscape editor is cautious but positive, with these words: As researchers gain a better understanding of the interactions between our nervous and immune systems, bioelectrical medicine is increasingly looking promising in treating numerous conditions, from pain to diabetes to possibly even cancer.

The idea is to target the same receptors as biochemical therapeutics; so, for example, pain relief electrotherapeutics will aim at deadening the nerves which transmit pain, much as analgesics do. It's a limited model but it's a good start!

Kevin Tracey, MD, President and CEO, The Feinstein Institute for Medical Research and Senior Vice President of Research, North Shore University Hospital, Manhasset, New York, explained to the doctors' newswire service "Medscape" about the potential of electricity-based therapy.

We had developed a new anti-inflammatory molecule, named CNI-1493, and we were studying its effects in the brain. Surprisingly, a small amount of CNI-1493 in the brain completely blocked the release of tumor necrosis factor (TNF)—a proinflammatory cytokine—throughout the body of the animal.

Turns out this CNI-1493 was acting by stimulating the vagus nerve, a very large cranial nerve that runs widely throughout the body, and is almost identical with parasympathetic function (parasympathetic means calm, relaxed, sleep, rest, inflammation quenched mode).

The results were completely unexpected and generated a series of papers in *Science* and *Nature* journals.

1. [Tracey KJ. The inflammatory reflex. Nature. 2002;420:853-859. Abstract

2. Wang H, Yu M, Ochani M, et al. Nicotinic acetylcholine receptor alpha7 subunit is an essential regulator of inflammation. Nature. 2003;421:384-388. Abstract

3. Rosas-Ballina M, Olofsson PS, Ochani M, et al. Acetylcholine-synthesizing T cells relay neural signals in a vagus nerve circuit. Science. 2011;334:98-101. Abstract

But why not stimulate the vagus nerve directly? Of course orthodoxy wants to do this with a HUGE intervention, implanting an electronic "buzz" device right on the nerve. It will cost $20,000 $30,000 and will need repeating every few years. A *perfect* money spinner! No wonder Glaxo-Smith-Kline was willing to invest $50 million into the research.

Indirect Vagus Nerve Stimulation

What, not heard of this? Where have you been living? Haha! Joking aside, it can seriously compete as one of the greatest advances in the early 21st century.

Well, the good news is that we can stimulate the vagus verve indirectly. An electrical current applied to the skin just upwards and inwards of the shoulder is easily picked up and acted on by this important nerve.

Almost any microcurrent therapy device can do this, if applied in exactly the right place. Bingo! The result is almost instant calming of inflammation and the ensuing benefits, from relaxation, reduced pain, improved sleep function or increased blood flow and cellular nutrition.

The vagus nerve, as you can see, the sensory network that tells the brain what's going on in our organs, most specially the digestive tract (stomach and intestines), lungs and heart, spleen, liver and kidneys, not to mention a range of other nerves that are involved in everything from talking to eye contact to facial expressions and even your ability to tune in to other people's voices. It is made of thousands upon thousands of fibers, operating far below the level of our conscious mind. It plays a vital role in sustaining overall wellness. It is an essential part of the parasympathetic nervous system, which is responsible for calming organs after the stressed "fight-or-flight" adrenaline response to danger. [https://www.meltmethod.com/blog/vagus-nerve/]

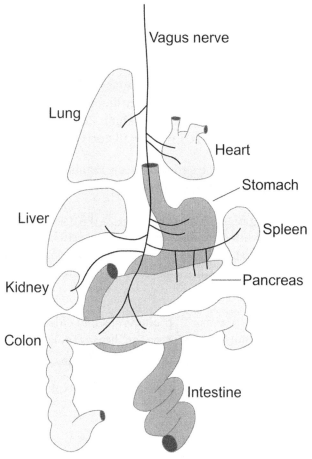

Vagus nerve

Lung

Heart

Stomach

Liver

Spleen

Kidney

Pancreas

Colon

Intestine

Access this video on YouTube, if you want to learn more:
https://www.youtube.com/watch?v=bNPfjLnnJzA [last accessed 23/9/2020]

Lullabies Still Work!

Even in this day and age of canned, background and streamed music, a gentle song works wonders at bedtime!

Every Mom, Sis and Nanny knows that a great way to get a child to sleep is to sing a lullaby. Science supports this common observation, showing that children of all ages, from premature infants to elementary school children, sleep better after listening to soothing melodies.

Soothing music should be a standard part of sleep hygiene.

OK, you may not want your Mom, Sis or spouse to sing to you at night. But these days there are numerous electronic devices to lull you to sleep! With streaming apps and portable speakers, it's easier than ever to take advantage of the power of music wherever you go. The right kind of music at bedtime can improve your ability to fall asleep quickly and feel more rested.

In one study, adults who listened to 45 minutes of music before going to sleep reported having better sleep quality beginning on the very first night. [Lai, H. L., & Good, M. (2005). Music improves sleep quality in older adults. Journal of advanced nursing, 49(3), 234–244. https://doi.org/10.1111/j.1365-2648.2004.03281.x]

It appears to be a cumulative thing. Listening to music regularly in bed before you fall asleep has better and better results through time.

It is noteworthy that listening to music can significantly decrease the time it takes to fall asleep. In a study of women with symptoms of insomnia, participants played a self-selected album when getting into bed for 10 consecutive nights. Before adding music to their evening routine it took participants from 27 to 69 minutes to fall asleep, after adding music it only took 6 to 13 minutes.

[Johnson J. E. (2003). The use of music to promote sleep in older women. Journal of community health nursing, 20(1), 27–35. https://doi.org/10.1207/S15327655JCHN2001_03]

Moreover, the quality of sleep is deeper and we all know how valuable that is.

How Does Music Effect Us?

Several studies suggest that music enhances sleep because of its effects on the regulation of hormones, including cortisol, the "stress hormone". Being stressed and having elevated levels of cortisol can increase alertness and lead to poor sleep. Listening to music on the other hand decreases levels of cortisol, which is good news and reason enough, all on its own!

Music also triggers the release of dopamine, a hormone released during pleasurable activities, like eating, exercise, and sex.

This release can boost good feelings at bedtime and address pain, another common cause of sleep issues. Physical and psychological responses to music are effective in reducing both acute and chronic physical pain.

[Chai, P. R., Carreiro, S., Ranney, M. L., Karanam, K., Ahtisaari, M., Edwards, R., Schreiber, K. L., Ben-Ghaly, L., Erickson, T. B., & Boyer, E. W. (2017). Music as an Adjunct to Opioid-Based Analgesia. Journal of medical toxicology, 13(3), 249–254]

Listening to the right sort of music can aid relaxation by soothing the autonomic nervous system. The autonomic nervous system is part of your body's natural system for controlling automatic or unconscious processes, including those within the heart, lungs, and digestive system. Music improves sleep through calming parts of the autonomic nervous system, leading to slower breathing, lower heart rate, and reduced blood pressure.

That's a ton of good reasons to go to sleep with a sweet serenade!

What Kind Of Music Is Best?

It is not within the remit of this book to tell you what to listen to, or help you create a sleep time playlist. It's mostly a matter of choice.

Avoid songs that cause strong emotional reactions: We all have songs that bring up strong emotions, such as sadness. Listening to those while trying to sleep may not be a great idea, so try music that's neutral or positive.

One thing I do know is that slow baroque music (like Vivaldi from the 17th century) has good science for creating calm and relaxation. I do not know what the rock and roll equivalent of that is. In fact rock and roll is not so good for sleep; ballads are better.

But there are two factors we can all agree on: a self-curated playlist (or one that has been designed specifically with sleep in mind) works best. Personal musical preferences seem to have the most effect on a person's physiology. That makes sense.

The other factor is tempo. Fast music tends to lift the spirits and enliven a person. That's the last thing we want at bedtime. For a full somnolent effect, a slow and gentle rhythm is good.

Music that is around 60-80 beats per minute works best. That's similar to the natural heart rate (60 – 100 beats per minute), which may be why it works.

If you don't want to create your own playlist, or don't know how, YouTube has thousands of hours of music to choose from. Look for videos categorized as "soothing", sleep or "relaxing" sounds, often coupled with the sound of waterfalls, the ocean waves, or gentle rain. Some relaxing music videos are 3 or 4 hours and upwards. That's more than enough to see you to sleep.

You can capture tracks as an audio MP3 and play that through your device. But DO NOT PUT THE PHONE OR TABLET NEXT TO YOUR HEAD. Use speakers located across the room instead.

Do you need extra help? Certified music therapists are professionals trained in using music to improve mental and physical health. A music therapist can assess a person's individual needs and create a treatment plan that can involve both listening to and creating music. For more information on music therapy, talk with your doctor or visit the American Music Therapy Association or the equivalent in other countries.

8. Energy Adjustments

Acupuncture certainly works. When I was professor at the university in Sri Lanka, I saw a man operated on with no other anesthetic than acupuncture needles at the right treatment points! A tumor the size of a soccer ball was removed from the side of his neck and face. He felt nothing, he said.

So why can't "adjusting the Ch'i", the flow of energies around the human body, have a beneficial effect?

Surprisingly, there is some science to support this. In 2021 *The Journal of Chinese Studies* published the results of a meta analysis. Researchers consulted seven medical databases and found twenty-four randomized controlled trials (RCTs) that compared acupuncture either pharmacotherapy or sham-acupuncture therapy. In the subsequent quantitative meta-analysis of studies comparing acupuncture versus pharmacotherapy, fifteen RCTs demonstrated that acupuncture had a significant effect on patients with insomnia as assessed by the Pittsburgh sleep quality index (PSQI)

These results suggest that insomnia patients may experience significant improvement in symptoms but this was only after more than three weeks of acupuncture treatment compared to pharmacological treatments.

Other ways of moving around energies in a beneficial way could include (depending on your view), Tai Ch'i, Yoga, massage and "hands on". Try them all!

Here I publish a very simple energy remedy I call sweeping...

Hands Sweeping Remedy

This is one I developed during experiments with my first wife Pauline, who was a very fine nurse. Working together, we found that using our hands to sweep over a person's body can make him or her feel better, calmer and more harmonious. It can even "sweep away" pain. It sets the stage for better, more relaxing sleep.

We theorized that it was about aligning turbulent energies around the person's body. The general rule in health and healing is that turbulence is bad, alignment (coherence) is good.

Have him or her lie on a bed, sofa or therapists couch. No degree of undress is required. Tell him or her to shut their eyes and relax.

Start with the person prone (face down) and work on the shoulders, back, buttocks and legs. Take both your hands and sweep along the body. Try to imagine they are covered in mud or jello and you are trying to wipe it away. That will give you the right sort of motion.

It is a sort of cleansing motion and it's a cleansing effect we are trying for.

Note this is a whole body technique. Don't just concentrate on a part. Turn him or her to the supine position (on their back) and repeat the whole process.

This remedy is quick: 10 – 15 minutes produces fast change; then it fades away. Not much to be gained by going on and on at it.

Applications: fatigue, upset, confusion, ailments, malaise, fever, tooth and jaw pain, earache, emotional storms, sickly part, discomfort short of pain and, of course, insomnia. It's also good for bellyache but you must remember the dangers of the "acute abdomen" (severe bellyache can denote serious, even life-threatening complaints).

[lightly edited from my *Supernoetics*® *Ex-Press* dated 23 March 2015: "The King Of All Communications"]

9. Psychological And Inner Deep Work

For the longest time, psychologists and psychiatrists have supposed that sleeplessness is just one of the symptoms of psychological disturbance. Wrong! It is emerging that sleeplessness is more often the cause than the result of problems.

In fact, it's a two-way street: sleep deprivation causes psychological issues and psychological disturbances can wreck sleep.

Matthew Walker, professor of neuroscience and psychology at the University of California, Berkeley says that "almost all psychiatric disorders show some problems with sleep." But, he says, scientists previously believed the psychiatric problems triggered the sleep issues. New research from his lab, however, suggests the reverse is the case; that is, sleep deprivation and sleep disturbance are causing some psychological disturbances. [https://www.scientificamerican.com/article/can-a-lack-of-sleep-cause/] By Nikhil Swaminathan on October 23, 2007

Chronic sleep problems affect 50% to 80% of patients in a typical psychiatric practice, compared with 10% to 18% of adults in the general population. Sleep problems are particularly common in patients with anxiety, depression, bipolar disorder, and attention deficit hyperactivity disorder (ADHD).

Studies using different methods and populations estimate that 65% to 90% of adult patients with major depression, and about 90% of children with this disorder, experience some kind of sleep problem. Most patients with depression have insomnia, but about one in five also suffer from obstructive sleep apnea.

In bipolar disorder, this can rise to nearly 100% of patient sleep badly. Studies in different populations report that 69% to 99% of patients experience insomnia or report less need for sleep during a manic episode. In bipolar depression, however, studies report that 23% to 78% of patients sleep excessively (hypersomnia), while others may experience insomnia or restless sleep.

The brain basis of a mutual relationship between sleep and mental health is not yet completely understood. But neuroimaging and neurochemistry studies suggest that a good night's sleep helps foster both mental and emotional resilience, while chronic sleep deprivation sets the stage for negative thinking and emotional vulnerability.

Key points

1. Sleep problems are more likely to affect patients with psychiatric disorders than people in the general population.

2. Sleep problems may increase risk for developing particular mental illnesses, as well as result from such disorders.

3. Treating the sleep disorder may help alleviate symptoms of the mental health problem.

What Are The Options?

This book is specifically written around the avoidance of sleep medications (drugs known as *"sleeping pills" and all related).*

For the psychological approach, start with relaxation techniques, meditation, guided imagery, deep breathing exercises, and progressive muscle relaxation (alternately tensing and releasing muscles), all of which can counter sleeplessness, anxiety and racing thoughts.

Because people with insomnia tend to worry and become preoccupied with not falling asleep, cognitive behavioral therapy (CBT) techniques help them to change negative expectations and try to build more confidence that they can have a good night's sleep. These techniques can also help to change the "blame game" of attributing every personal problem during the day on lack of sleep.

Hypnotherapy

Possibly the most profound psychological intervention is that of hypnotherapy. I have several friends who are top hypnotherapists in the world and they say it IS effective and the usual baloney bandied around by critics, that hypnotism is self-delusion or a hoax, is just plain wrong.

According to hypnotherapy expert Elaine Kissel, anyone having difficulty sleeping tends to become more stressed and apprehensive about another night of missed or un-restful, even interrupted sleep cycles. This of course aggravates the issues and sets the person up for another difficult night. So hypnosis, which is a powerful tool, can be employed to help people relax and stop worrying so much about being able to sleep.

Dr Kissel works with people over the world with her Whole Mind Hypnotherapy system. She created the famous *Mind Mastery* course, and has authored several pertinent books: "*The Mind Is Willing,*" "*The Addiction Dilemma and Solutions,*" and "*Set Backs and Come Backs: How To Overcome Stuck States.*"

According to her, there are many issues that cause sleep problems, beside neurological problems. Some are simply poor sleep habits, which means not setting and maintaining a regular bedtime schedule, etc. (sleep hygiene, p. 16). Also stress, worry, trying too hard to sleep, not being able to relax and quiet their minds keeps people in an awake state. Fear of nightmares and having night time pain, depression, anxiety etc. All are interfering with the natural mind/brain biological circadian rhythms that enable sleep to occur.

Hypnosis when used well can eliminate all of those issues and reestablish healthy sleep patterns. Hypnosis is also a tool to enable us to explore the causes of the sleep disorder and resolve them at the root level.

Though honestly Mind Mastery has helped countless people overcome sleep problems without my hypnotherapy or the self-hypnosis training course I have created.

Dr. Kissel always recommends her clients and students to not to try to sleep. In order to sleep we must let go, consciously. Most people don't know how to do that. People need to know about the mind body/conscious and subconscious relationship; unfortunately that is often not a healthy one. It's important bring about a much more positive relationship. That's why hypnosis, when used properly is a wonderful tool to facilitate positive changes.

Hypnosis isn't just relaxing the mind; it relaxes the body, and brings about inner calm, peaceful emotional states, too. It can be used to create positive inner experiences because it relaxes that busy body conscious mind and enables us to access the subconscious and all its powerful resources, and employ them to our advantage. Improving quantity and quality of sleep is just one of its countless benefits.

There are myriad levels/states of hypnosis. Everyone can be hypnotized, when the right methods are employed for each individual. As in most cases, there is no one size fits all method of inducing this altered state of consciousness, or employing it effectively in each case. That's where the practitioners expertise comes in.

Day dreaming, or mind wandering, is often a daily habit for many, which is actually drifting into hypnosis.

Sleep studies have proven that hypnotic states are those very brief brain changes that initiate the sleep processes. So inducing hypnosis is a very natural way to facilitate the sleep cycle. And everyone can learn self-hypnosis techniques and how to employ them to go to sleep and sleep well. It's a natural, safe and easy way to develop healthy sleep habits and many other life improving changes.

Dr. Kissel can be contacted at: +1 (248) 595 1010 email: kyhpno@aol.com and her website is: www.kisselhypnosis.com

If you don't have ready access to a practitioner, my friend John Farley tells us that the easiest way to utilize hypnosis is by listening to a sleep hypnosis audio before bedtime. Of course, learning to self-hypnotize is a useful skill that you can take anywhere and use anytime.

Neuro-Linguistic Programming

Another way to deliberately alter what's going on in a person's mind and give them control over it is neuro-linguistic programming (NLP). There is no room in this manual to teach NLP. But it's specifically about altering meta-programs: tiny little runs of thoughts and ideas that start in one place and end up in another; often somewhere the client does NOT want to be, with thoughts or behaviors that are disempowering!

If you suffer with insomnia, what exactly is going on in your mind just before you go to sleep? "I suppose tonight will be bad again," and thoughts like that do not set you up well for sleep!

If your problem is severe and causing excessive health damage, you may want to seek out the help of an NLP practitioner. As with all such, there are good ones and bad ones! But you could start the quest on your own.

Nicole Schneider wrote an interesting piece for the Global NLP Training website (globalnlptraining.com), in which she suggest the following little catechism:

1. What time do you specifically wake? Is it a simple matter that you wake up too late, and therefore cannot go to bed on time?

2. What activities in your day cause you stress and an "unhealthy" adrenaline push? What specifically could you do to change this?

3. What would happen if you changed the way you do these activities?

4. Who is giving you stress? What specifically could you do to change this? What would happen if you stopped seeing this person, or changed the way you perceive them? Is there work needed on a personal evolution level?

5. How much coffee, tea, and/or other caffeinated drinks do you drink? At what time of day? Can something be reduced here, or consumed at an earlier time?

6. Do you eat a lot of food late at night? Consider eating earlier.

7. What specifically do you do to relax? And what would happen if you created more relaxing points in your day?

8. Between 4 PM and the time you go to bed, what activities do you do? Do they involve a lot of electronics, especially close to bedtime?

9. What would happen if you created a "before bed" routine?

10. What specifically do you think about before you go to bed?

The last is an important key. People often can't sleep because they are thinking about things that stress them out. It is amazing how it is outside of conscious awareness that these thoughts don't just happen to a person. Any NLP practitioner knows that when the brain can't help itself, it will randomly start working on its own. The brain needs a little help from its owner. Instead of thinking about things that are unpleasant, or require a lot mental activity, think about things that relax you and/or things that make you happy.

[https://www.globalnlptraining.com/blog/nlp-better-sleep/]

That's probably why gratitude—and specifically keeping a gratitude journal—is so helpful for sleep. It focuses you intently on the good things in your life, to the exclusion of worries and cares. So keeping a nightly gratitude journal is also good sleep hygiene.

10. The Desperation Remedy

It's tough but it WILL work! It's very simple. When bedtime is looming you go for a long walk... and then some!

The way to do this is to walk away from home until you feel really tired. Then you turn around and walk back home. That should fix it!

Of course that's a laborious technique. But you wouldn't have to do it more than a few times. It need not—should not—be used as a routine. Just a last ditch sleep aid.

But don't forget, regular vigorous physical activity is good for sleep in general. Ask anyone who has been on a sailing holiday, spent a few weeks on a kibbutz or walked the pilgrimage route to Santiago de Compostela!

Regular aerobic activity has also been found to help people fall asleep faster, spend more time in deep sleep, and awaken less often during the night.

Even gardening can be a great sleep remedy, if you keep at it till you feel tired!

Part 3. Tips For Coming Off Sleep Medications

Most sleep drugs are supposed to be for temporary use; at least that's what it says on the label insert. But most doctors ignore this point and may go on prescribing sleep medication to the same patient for months, or even years.

Sleeping pills and sedatives can have very strong side effects, including problems with memory or concentration, drowsiness, muscle weakness, abnormal behavior and sleep disorders. They can also affect people's ability to drive and, particularly in older and unwell people, increase the likelihood of falling.

One way to stop sleep medication is just go cold turkey but if your doctor has been naughty, prescribing heavy medications for sleep, such as SSRIs (Prozac, Zoloft, Paxil, etc.), Benzodiazepines (Valium, Halcion, Restoril), or tricyclic antidepressants, such as amitriptyline, this is not an option. Don't try it. It may trigger seizures.

Instead, you need to taper off.

- For the first two weeks, take half of your usual nightly dose.
- When week three occurs, cut your dosage in half again. …
- Continue that dose through week four.
- Keeping with that same dose, switch to taking it once every second night and then every third night, instead of every night of the week.

You can always stay on a dose for a longer period, until you feel comfortable and ready to take the next step in reducing the dose.

Experts say it is best to take 2 – 4 months to come off heavy sleep or tranquillizer medications.

If not done carefully or too abruptly, you may get a rebound withdrawal response that keeps you from sleeping well. Depending on the specific drug, symptoms can start within a few hours, but they may also be delayed, sometimes occurring even weeks after use has been discontinued. Typical symptoms of withdrawal include trouble sleeping, restlessness, anxiety, shivering or circulation problems. They're similar to the symptoms that were originally targeted when using the sedative. We call this rebound insomnia.

"If you stop too quickly you can get rebound insomnia, which makes symptoms worse," says sleep expert Dr. Lawrence Epstein, an instructor in medicine at Harvard Medical

School. [https://www.health.harvard.edu/staying-healthy/the-savvy-sleeper-wean-yourself-off-sleep-aids]

Rebound insomnia then convinces users they need the drugs to sleep. In reality, the medication is just preventing withdrawal symptoms. That cycle creates dependence, which is different from an addiction that's characterized by compulsive use and preoccupation with a drug that interferes with normal life.

Other Help For Getting Off Sleep Medications

- cognitive behavior therapy (CBT), which helps you redirect your thoughts to reduce anxiety about sleeping. A number of moderate quality studies support the idea that more people stop taking sedatives when they have psychological support. [https://pubmed.ncbi.nlm.nih.gov/26106751]

- hypnotherapy. Elaine Kissel (p. 42) reassures us that hypnosis has the added benefit that it can be used to help an individual withdraw comfortably from doctor-prescribed sleep meds and store bought sleeping aids and allow him or her to develop healthy natural sleep patterns.

- relaxation techniques such as guided visualization

- recognizing the stimuli that prevent sleep, such as television, computer, or smartphone screens

- improving sleep hygiene, by using the bed for sleep and sex only; blocking as much noise and light as possible; going to bed and waking at the same times each day; and getting out of bed if you haven't fallen asleep within 20 minutes

- dietary changes, such as avoiding alcohol, caffeine, and foods that promote acid indigestion.

It's tough to get off medication but you have enough options here in this manual to find one or more suitable alternative to long-term or permanent medication, with all the attendant side-effects.

You will sleep better in the end, I promise, if you can dump medication and use a natural remedy instead.

Good luck and sweet dreams!

Made in the USA
Monee, IL
21 August 2021